THE SECRET OF BEING SLIM & FIT IN 5 WORDS

Alexa Woodgate

Introduction

Why has this book the title: The secret of being slim & fit in 5 words? The answer is simple: If you act in the way I tell you, you will be slim & fit. Surley!

I

promise

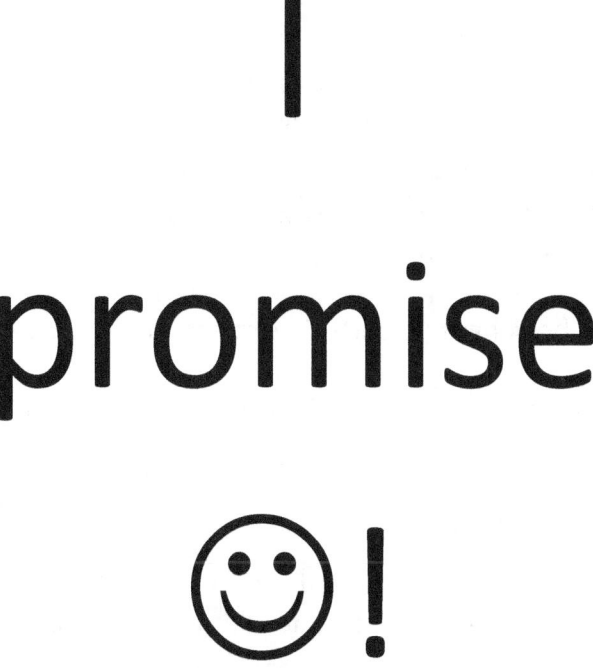

!

Every time I looked in a magazin with stars, famous people and celebrities I had one problem:

I felt too fat.

And every time I saw a sporty person I had another problem:

I thought I was not fit enough.

But this time is nowadays more than 10 years away. It´s history.

The first point is: I have recognized, that I must not be perfect. I must not reach 10 points of 10 points. 8 points are enough. With this 8 points you are slimmer and fitter than 80% of the other people. But you only need 50 % and not 200 % to reach your aims.

This book has two parts: The question of lesson 1 is:

How can I loose weight and become as slim I want to be?

I want that you read this book. I will not give you the first secret of being slim (It´s only two words.) on the hand. You have to search for this two words in lesson 1. If you read the whole text (It is a simple and short, easy to understand text.) you will find this two words. To make you sure, that you have found them behind this two words appears the word: secret.

Lesson 2 has also only one question:

What must I do for getting fit?

I told you before: You must only reach 80%. Together with your slim figure it will show maximum effect. I will tell you this secret after reading the short and simple text in Lesson 2. Again you will read the word secret when you reach the aim. This secret is built up by only 3 words.

Only 2 lessons, only 5 simple words. I tell you: If you do the way I want you to:

You will be slim & fit ☺!

You only must do want I want you to do.

You will loose weight.

In 6 months you are fitter than ever. In 2 years you will reach the highscore. But remember: 80% are enough.

Congrets: You are on the right way!

Let´s start with lesson 1....

Lesson 1: Loose your fat

There are a few new diets. They are not so bad.

One is the 6:1 diet. This means: 6 days a week you eat not too much.

And 1 day a week you can eat what you want. I like this diet, because you can eat what you want:

Cake, muffins, donuts ☺

Ice-cream, cookies, chocolate ☺

But only at one day a week. The rest of the week: Be disciplined. Do not eat more than 1.500 calories. If you drink alcohol the calories must be added.

In the first weeks people normally eat very much at the day everything is allowed. But after a few weeks the hunger and appetite gets smaller. So they eat not so much.

This is the reason why this diet is effective:

You loose your hunger.

So after a few weeks it is not hard for you to eat lesser. Your hunger decreases and you do not miss the cookies, donuts and muffins. You eat one of them and you feel so filled up that you do not want to eat another one.

This is like you smoke a lot of cigarettes and after a few weeks training you don´t miss them.

So I can tell you:

The 6:1 diet... works ☺!

The other one I mentioned above is the 3:2 diet. For 3 days you only eat up to 900 calories. The following 2 days it is:

All you can eat! ☺

Similar to the 6:1 diet in the first weeks people eat during this 2 days very much. But after a few weeks they don´t want. In their body and mind a metamorphosis takes place:

They stop eating to feel happy. They stop eating to have the feeling of a full stomach. They don´t try to get more adventure in their life by eating.

Why?

If you do not eat much your body has more energy.

If you have more energy you can do all the things you want to. And then?

You forget to eat and eat and eat...

In this way you can fulfill your dreams. Stop wasting your energy with eating.

Make your dreams come true instead! Find yourself a new partner. Live your dreams. Be happy.

And when you are happy, you don´t need to eat to feel happy.

So remember:

The 6:1 and the 3:2 diet are good methods.

But this is not the secret. The secret is another. Later more...

Why is it so difficult to loose fat?

Here is the **truth**:

- ✓ Women have normally less muscles than men. So for women it is harder to loose fat. Muscles burn the fat. If you have less muscles you have to eat less. Sorry ☹

- ✓ When you get older you need less calories. Most people eat like they are teenager. The older you are you must have a great discipline to eat not too much. Your body doesn´t need a lot of calories. Sorry ☹

✓ Normally the truth is: Everything that tastes good, has too much calories. If you love some kind of food very much, it has much to much calories. The better it tastes the more bad it is for you. Sorry ☹ **but**

This is only for the first few weeks right. If you have changed your style of eating your body will change. And you will change:

You will love the things you hated.
Believe me: You will love vegetables. You will feel bad when you eat noodles or pizza. Or white bread.

✓ You need to make sport. The formula is simple:

First: Eat less calories!

Second: Move, make sport!

✓ Look at slim & fit people. Normally you need 10 persons to find one, which is slim & fit.
✓ 9 of 10 Persons, who are slim & fit are young or look young.

So, if you are old make sports and you look young.
☺
If you are young: Keep on doing sports for staying

young. Conserve your youth.

And now: A little bit mathematics:

Your age, your gender, your quantity of muscles and your movement define how much calories you need a day.

Too much calories = fat and flabby body ☹

Normally you need around 1.500 to 2000 calories a day. NOT MORE!!!!

Think: Nuts, donuts, sweeties have all around 600 to 800 calories / 100 g.

So you can drink two bottles of beer, eat two sandwiches with chocolate cream and some noodles: Result: You are hungry and has eaten the calories you are allowed to eat at one day.

Fuck! This is really not much.

Remember: Two bottles of beer & two sandwiches with chocolate cream & only a few noodles

=

all calories for one day ☹!!!

So: You must look for goods with less calories!!!!

If you like to drink beer...it is ok. But the calories of the beer you must spare.

Every day one cupcake = 250 Calories.

1 Cupcake a day in one year = 250 Calories x 365 = > 90.000 calories!!

If you live your normal life without this daily cupcake you can loose > 9 kg each year!!!!!!!!!!!!!!!!!!!!!!!!!!!!!!!!!! (10.000 calories a needed for 1 kilo body fat).

Remember this simple example! You must not starve hunger to get slim. You only need a little bit of discipline ☺.

Let´s make this deal: In the first week of your new life you eat per week 1 cupcake less. In the following 1 more less. You must continue in this way, until you only eat 1 cupcake a week. This is in the spirit of the 6:1 diet, I´ve mentioned above.

Be smart & clever ☺!

The magic three

The secret is: Avoid Carbohydrates (Secret!)

What does a healthy person need to eat?

?

Carbohydrates, Protein, Fat.

These are the three ingredients. Not more.

In former days there was this GOLDEN rule:

50 % Carbohydrates
40 % Protein
10 % Fat.

In nowadays this is wrong!!!

In former days people worked hard. Very hard. Only a few machines helped the mankind. So they had to take shovel & hammer and work very hard with their bodies. There were less cars. So a lot of people drove with their bicycle, if they had one.

Lots of people had to go by foot. They were moving all the day. To the work, on the job, after work. There was no TV to look on in the evening.

Those people were very busy. Farmers had to work very hard too. Women had to work at the job and at home very hard. No washing-machine, no electric iron, no help.....

So: People in former time needed carbohydrates. They give the body energy to work hard. But there was only hard work and often not enough carbohydrates. Bread was very expensive. So they had to eat vegetables and fruits.

And in present?

On every corner you can find a bakery with cheap bread.

Go to the next bakery and look to those people, who are eating bread in the morning. Most of them are too thick. They eat tons of sandwiches.

Attention: Sandwiches make you fat!!!

You must avoid bread. Maybe today you eat bread 7 days a week. Try to eat less.

In the beginning it is hard. But try it!!!!!!

After a few days it is getting easier. And you will have more energy than ever. You will not be tired after eating.

Try it!

Try it!
Your aim is: Only three times a week bread.

Try it. After a few weeks your hunger for bread is getting **smaller** and smaller and smaller....

And your hips are getting smaller and smaller and smaller and smaller!

Another great enemy are….

What do you think?

????????????????

Beware of the enemies

Okay, I give you the answer:

Noodles.

Fat people love noodles. With sausage.

Never ever eat noodles in the evening! :-/

It is like eating bread. Your stomach is full, you are satisfied and tired.

But:

You are no baby.

You don´t need to feel satisfied with full stomach like a baby.

Noodles not more than one time a week.

Remember:

Noodles not more than one time a week!!!

Better:
No noodles. Less bread.

Remember.

No noodles. Less bread.

Your aim is: Only 30 % carbohydrates.

Why?

You do not need more.

Why?

You are a modern person. You have a car. You have no hard work for your body.

You are no baby. You do not need to be satisfied and tired.

YOU ARE NO BABY!!!

All fat people eat to much bread!

And you don´t need much bread.

Only three times a week.

No noodles in the evening.

The next point is:

Eat fat.

But not too much.

But: You need fat. Your body needs it.

My doctor told me from women, who didn´t do so.

She was depressed. If you don´t like to be depressed, you must eat fat.

But not too much! Only a little bit. Fat is very dangerous for your figure and for your health.

The problem is: The evolution learned your body to eat as much fat as he can. In historic times when mankind were hunters and gatherers it was very important to do so for not to starve. Only time by time when hunters had slayed an animal they could eat a little bit of fat. So every time they could eat fat they had to eat fat.

Today the situation is for most people completely different. There is such an opulence of foods. And creamy, fatty, oily foods.

So you must be tough. Eat fat but eat **only a bit** fat.

And remember the first secret (2 of 5 words):

Avoid Carbohydrates.

Lesson 2: Fit & Slender

What kind of sport is most effective to get fit & slender?

The top ten are:

1. Martial Arts

2. Cycling

3. Athletics

4. Rowing

5. Figure skating

6. (Beach)-Volleyball

7. Badminton

8. Tennis

9. Football

10. Swimming

In many magazines you can read headlines like this

Shape your body in 5 weeks!

You can get a beach body in 2 weeks!

Forever fit & slender!

Get your sixpack in only 14 days!

Do you know this? You see these magazines and you think: "Wow! Fine!". You buy this magazine. You read the article. And you must recognize they are writing bullshit.

Believe me: To become fit & slender you must work on it for years.

Not 20 ore 10 years.

It is 5 years if you do it step by step.

You much sports a day?

If you really do one of the top ten I´ve mentioned above you have to do it 2 to 3 times a week.

Be careful!

Start with only 1 time the week. This is very important. After a half year you can make it 2 times a week. And after 2 years 3 times week.

Many people make the mistake to start too fast. Years and years they make no sport and from one day to the other they want to make every day sport.

This is wrong. You will loose your motivation very soon. You will get hurt because your body has slowly to adept to your choosen sport.

I make martial arts since 20 years. So much people came into the course. After the first lesson they were enthusiastic. They said: "This is my new life. I will make this sport every day for the rest of my life." Next day you can see them in the course. Next day too.

But:

After 2 weeks, longest 2 month you never ever see those people again. They loose their motivation because their body says: STOP!!!! This is too much in this short time!

So..the best solution is:

START SLOWLY. Create a solid foundation.

Choose the sport you like. You must forget the time while you are doing it.

In most gyms there are people with serious faces. Without a smile. They do not have fun. They make sports because they think they must do it.

But this is wrong. Make sports while having fun.

For me it´s better to have interaction with other people while doing sports.

Think about: What kind of sport do you like? Which kind of sports makes you forget the time while you are doing it?

This is the right kind of sport for you.

Avoid sports you do not like

and which is boring you.

The second secret is:

Make 100 push-up each day!!!

This is all to get find & slender. Maybe you think 100 is too much. But you are wrong.

First week: 10 push-up each day.

Second week: 20 push-up each day

Third week: 30 push-up each day

And so on.

Start slowly with 10 push up each day.

Push-ups are great for your muscles all over your body.

They are good for your back. They will help you against back pain.

Many people´ back look like an (

Their shoulders hang. They have no tension in their body.

Believe me:

After a few month with 100 push up each day you have tension in your body.

Imagine:

You eat less carbohydrates (first secret)

and make 100 push up each day (second secret).

Remember the secret of

BEING SLIM & FIT IN 5 WORDS

is:

Avoid carbohydrates

&

100 push-up/day.

In best case you ad:

✓ two to three times a week your favorite sport

✓ it would be good if your favorite sport is part of the top ten list I have mentioned above

✓ avoid carbohydrates

✓ one day a week you are allowed to eat what you want

✓ after each 100 days you can make one week the following things:

✓ eat what you want

✓ make no sports.

So many people say: Tomorrow I change my life completely. But this is the wrong way.

24:

You must go step by step. And every week you must rest for one day. This is the best solution.

Lesson 3: Mental help

At the end here is some mental help for you:

✓ Do not give up, if you are not consequent for a week or a month.

✓ You only have to restart. Again and again. The you reach your aim.

✓ Try meditation and other mental help. This will help you to feel yourself better in your body and life.

I wish you all the best. Love yourself.